POCKET H

Ka

RELAX YOUR MUSCLES & MIND

Stephanie Pedersen

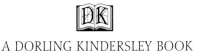

A DORLING KINDERSLEY BOOK

CONTENTS

HERBAL HISTORY

L ong before over-the-counter medications and prescription drugs came on the scene, herbs proved to be powerful healers. Every culture on earth has used herbal medicine. In fact, herbal usage is older than recorded history itself: herbal preparations have been found at the burial site of a Neanderthal man who lived over 60,000 years ago.

When it comes to herbal medicine, many healing systems are available and useful. Perhaps the best known are ayurveda, Chinese medicine, and Western herbalism. Ayurveda is a system of diagnosis and treatment that uses herbs in conjunction with breathing, meditation, and yoga. It has been practised in India for more than 2,500 years. Ayurveda gets its name from the Sanskrit words *ayuh*, meaning "longevity", and *veda*, meaning "knowledge". Indeed, in ayurvedic healing, health can be achieved only after identifying a person's physical and mental characteristics (called "dosha"). Then the proper preventative or therapeutic remedies are prescribed to help an individual maintain doshic balance.

OTHER HERBAL HEALING SYSTEMS

Chinese medicine is another healing system that uses herbs in combination with acupressure, acupuncture, and qi gong. Sometimes called traditional Chinese medicine (TCM), this ancient system is thought to be rooted as far back as 2,800BC in the time of emperor Sheng Nung. Known as China's patron saint of herbal medicine, Sheng Nung is credited as being among the first proponents of healing plants. Chinese medicine attempts to help the body correct energy imbalances. Therefore herbs are classified according to certain active characteristics, such as heating, cooling, moisturizing, or drying, and prescribed according to how they influence the activity of various organ systems.

Many herbal practitioners believe that Western herbalism can trace its roots to the ancient Sumerians, who – according to a medicinal recipe dating from 3,000BC – boasted a refined knowledge of herbal medicine. Records from subsequent cultures, such as the Assyrians, Egyptians, Israelites, Greeks, and Romans, show similar herbal healing systems. But these peoples weren't the only ones using beneficial plants. The Celts, Gauls, Scandinavians, and other early European tribes also healed with herbs. In fact, it was their knowledge, combined with the medicine brought by invading Moors and Romans, that formed the foundation for Western herbalism. Simply put, this foundation formed a comprehensive system wherein herbs were grouped according to how they affected both the body and specific body systems.

After the discovery of the New World, Western herbalism was refined further with the benefit of wisdom gained from the American Indians, and the routine use of herbal remedies by physicians and for domestic use can be traced as far back as the 1600s. Herbs also featured heavily in medical pharmacopoeia until the 1900s.

However, with the creation of synthetic medicines in the 1930s interest in herbal medicines began to wane. New drugs were the great white hope for a disease-free future, but as time has passed they have been found to cause as many problems in terms of side-effects and contraindications as they solve.

Now, throughout Europe, America, and the world, gentler herbal remedies are enjoying a revival. What's been even more exciting is that many of the "folk" uses of these remedies have now been proven by science.

WHAT IS KAVA?

Kava is becoming increasingly popular, yet it is no medicinal newcomer – the herb boasts a long, distinguished history as an anti-anxiety medication, antidepressant, and sleep aid. In fact, kava has been used in Papua New Guinea, the Micronesian Islands, Fiji, Samoa, Tonga, Wallis, Vanuatu, Tahiti, and Hawaii for over 3,000 years – brewed into a drink to calm the nerves, increase libido, and promote sociability, and as a topical poultice to numb muscle aches. The kava plant is a hardy, flowering shrub belonging to the pepper family. Although 20 species of kava grow throughout the South Pacific, the Piper methysticum is the variety used medicinally. The plant, which reaches maturity from three to five years after planting, features pretty, heart-shaped leaves and can reach heights of three metres (10ft).

Although it isn't known who first used kava, the herb's usage predates Oceanic written history. The plant may have originated in New Guinea or Indonesia. It was spread, along with other plants (including sugar cane), from island to island by early Polynesian explorers. Each culture has its own story on the origins of kava. One Samoan story tells of a young woman who went to Fiji to marry a great chief. After a few years she decided to return home to Samoa. As she was getting ready to leave Fiji, she noticed a plant growing on a hill. After watching a feeble rat chewing on the plant become bold, strong, and energetic, she decided to take the plant (kava) back to Samoa. The plant thrived and reproduced in Samoa and soon, the Samoans were using its roots to trade with other islanders.

One tale from Tonga centres around a chief and a god, the chief taking the role of the servant, and the god taking the role of the chief. The chief had to serve a feast to a god but because it was a time of famine, he couldn't find any food. So the chief killed his only daughter and cooked her. The god immediately recognized human flesh, told the chief to bury his daughter's remains, and asked him to bring the plant that grew from that spot. When the chief presented the plant, the god showed him how to prepare a ceremonial drink from it.

On the small island of Manu'a islanders attribute kava to a god named Tangaloa. One day, Tangaloa visited earth on a fishing trip. At the end of the day, he wanted some kava drink to have with the fish he caught. Unfortunately, Tangaloa forgot to bring his kava with him, so he sent two mortals to heaven to bring him a root. Having never seen a kava root, they mistakenly brought the whole plant. As the god separated the roots from the plant, he scattered kava leaves, stems, flowers, and seeds all across the land; new kava plants sprouted wherever those parts fell.

By the 1700s, when the first European explorers arrived, kava was widely used throughout the Pacific region. Islanders showed their visitors how to use kava beverages for headaches, stress, and insomnia. Indeed, along with its sedative qualities, the herb's analgesic properties made it a popular medicinal aid before pharmaceutical painkillers existed. Kava's most important active components are known collectively as kavalactones. These include demthyoxyyangonin, dihydrokavain, yangonin, kavain, dihydromethysticin, and methysticin. Other constituents are simple sugars, protein, and potassium. It is in kava's mangled mass of root stock that the greatest concentration of these medicinal ingredients resides.

· ALTERNATIVE NAMES ·

Like many herbs, Kava is known by several names:

- ◆ Ava
- ◆ Awa Awa
- ◆ Gea
- ◆ Kava Kava
- ◆ Intoxicating Pepper
- ◆ Piper Methysticum
- ◆ Tonga

HERBAL FORMULATIONS

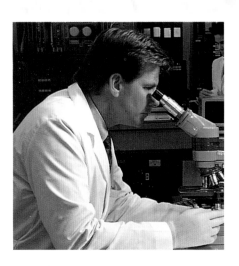

Researchers today perform thousands of rigorous clinical trials on the herbs sold in pharmacies and health stores. Most scientific studies with successful outcomes have used "standardized" herb formulations but the holistic approach is also currently finding favour. Standardized herb formulations means that particular therapeutic components are always present at specific concentrations. The benefit of standardization is that you will always be guaranteed a given potency but depending upon the method used to standardize, the full spectrum of constituents originally found in the herb might not be present in the final formulation. If all the components are present they are unlikely to be there in exactly the same proportions.

THE HOLISTIC APPROACH

Holistic herbal formulations, usually tinctures, contain the whole herb and their chemical composition will be as close as possible to the plant they derive from. Whole herb formulations may not always contain a consistent amount of active ingredients but manufacturers argue that it is the whole spectrum of ingredients, not just one or two active constituents, that determines the overall efficacy of the formulation. For advice on the most effective way to take specific herbs talk to a herbalist or pharmacist, or go to a reputable health store.

DO YOU HAVE A CONTRAINDICATION?

A contraindication is a common medical term that refers to a symptom or condition that makes a particular treatment inadvisable. For example, because kava has been shown to worsen Parkinson's disease symptoms, Parkinson's disease is a contraindication.

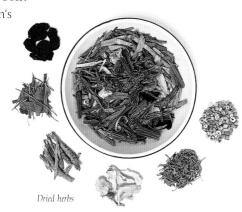

Dried herbs

· HERBAL BASICS ·

◆ Always follow the instructions on the label. Take the herb regularly and do not overdose.

◆ Don't expect instantaneous results. Some herbs may take a period of time to work.

◆ If you are pregnant don't take herbs without first seeking specific medical advice.

◆ Always check with your doctor if you are concerned that a herb may interact with a particular medication or be contraindicated by illness.

COMMON SIDE EFFECTS

Just like many medicinal herbs, kava can cause mild side effects, so take care:

DROWSINESS A small number of people experience drowsiness when taking kava, especially if they take it in large doses. For this reason avoid taking kava before driving or operating heavy machinery.

REDDENED EYES Some reports have linked kava with reddened eyes and more serious problems such as blood in the urine, blurred vision, shortness of breath, and yellowness of the skin. But these effects are only usually seen with truly massive doses of kava, and are unlikely in people taking normal amounts.

· PRECAUTIONS ·

◆ Kava should not be consumed with alcoholic drinks or other central nervous system depressants.

◆ Do not take kava if you are currently taking prescription medication for depression or anxiety. The effects of these drugs can be increased to potentially dangerous levels if taken with kava.

◆ The doses in this book are generally aimed at adults. We strongly suggest consulting a health professional before administering kava to a child.

◆ Kava should not be taken by individuals with Parkinson's disease; the herb worsens disease symptoms.

◆ Kava should not be taken by women who are pregnant, trying to conceive, or nursing.

◆ To avoid dangerous interactions between prescription medication and herbal medicine, individuals with AIDS, cancer, a connective tissue disease, heart disease, kidney disease, liver disease, tuberculosis, or any other chronic illness should consult their physician before using any herb.

Herbal supplements

FORMULA GUIDE

Herbal remedies are sold in many different forms. Listed below are some of the most common products:

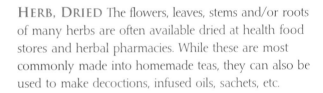

CAPSULES Capsules are usually made with gelatin and can be hard (made of two pieces, usually containing powders), or pliable (soft) and filled with liquid or paste. Two-piece capsules can also be pulled apart and the powder taken separately. Capsules usually contain fewer excipients (non-active) ingredients than tablets.

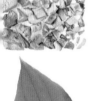

HERB, DRIED The flowers, leaves, stems and/or roots of many herbs are often available dried at health food stores and herbal pharmacies. While these are most commonly made into homemade teas, they can also be used to make decoctions, infused oils, sachets, etc.

HERB, FRESH Herbs used in culinary and medicinal ways (such as parsley or dill) are most often found fresh. These can be made into homemade extract, juice, infused oil, tea, and more.

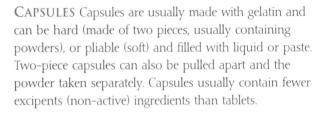

LIQUID EXTRACT (also called Extract). Macerated plant material is steeped over a period of time in a solvent or solvents such as alcohol, glycerin and/or water. The steeped liquid is then reduced to lessen the concentration of (or entirely remove) the solvents. Generally stronger than a tincture.

OIL, ESSENTIAL (also called Oil). Essential oils are the volatile oily components of herbs. They are found in tiny glands located in the flowers, leaves, roots and/ or bark and are mechanically or chemically extracted. They are prescribed almost exclusively for external use.

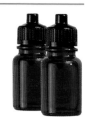

OINTMENTS Dried or fresh herbs are steeped in a base of oils and emulsifiers (such as beeswax, petroleum jelly or soft paraffin wax). After a period of time, the herbs are removed and the ointment packaged. For external use only.

SYRUPS Syrups are generally a combination of herbal extracts and a sweetener, such as honey or sugar. Generally used for colds, flu, and sore throats.

TABLETS Tablets are made of all the relevant herbal and tabletting aids compressed using very high pressure. They are also relatively less expensive than comparable hard and soft gelatin capsules. Chewable tablets may be used for adult or child formulations.

TEAS/INFUSIONS Commercial herbal tea bags, loose dried, or fresh herbs are all available. This is a pleasant and acceptable way to take a herb, although to digest a useful quantity of the herb several cups have to be drunk daily.

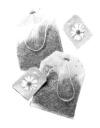

TINCTURES Tinctures are made by soaking plant material in a solvent – almost always alcohol – which is then pressed. Liquid from this pressing may be diluted with water before being packaged. Tinctures are an easy and pure way to take the herb.

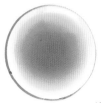

DYSMENORRHOEA

SYMPTOMS Mild to moderate pain during menstruation is normal and occurs when the uterus contracts to shed its temporary lining. However, sometimes the uterus contracts more than necessary, causing extreme pain. This condition is called dysmenorrhoea. It is believed to be caused by excessive levels of prostaglandins. The primary symptom is strong to severe pain in the lower abdomen during menstruation; this pain may radiate to the hips, buttocks, or thighs. Other signs include diarrhoea, dizziness, excessive perspiration, fatigue, nausea, and vomiting.

HOW KAVA CAN HELP Kava is an ideal menstrual aid, thanks to its ability to relax cramped uterine muscles. The herb also boasts analgesic powers that deaden severe uterine pain. Furthermore, kava's mood-improving and sedating powers help calm the fear and anxiety that dysmenorrhoea often causes.

Note: *Painful periods are not always a sign of dysmenorrhoea. In some cases they signal an underlying disease, such as endometriosis. If you suffer from painful periods, please see your doctor to rule out any existing illness.*

DOSAGES At the first sign of symptoms, enjoy 1 or 2 cups of kava tea, or for stronger relief take 250mg extract three times daily. A relaxing kava bath is also helpful. To a warm bath, add a teaspoon of kava tincture, or ½ teaspoon of essential oil.

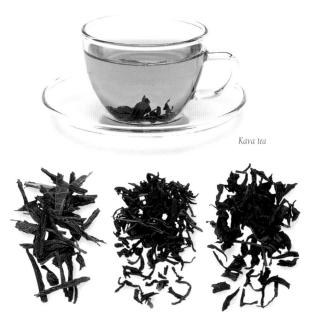

Kava tea

Dried kava

MENOPAUSAL SYMPTOMS

SYMPTOMS Menopause is not an illness but a natural condition that occurs when the ovaries no longer produce enough oestrogen to stimulate the lining of the uterus and vagina sufficiently. Simply put, menopause is when women no longer menstruate or get pregnant. It generally occurs somewhere between the ages of 40 and 60. One of the most famous signs of menopause is the hot flush, a sudden reddening of the face accompanied by a feeling of intense warmth. Other common symptoms include depressed mood, fluid retention, insomnia, irritability nervousness, night sweats, painful intercourse, rapid heart beat, susceptibility to bladder problems, thinning of vaginal tissues, vaginal dryness, and weight gain. It should be noted that some women experience few symptoms, while still others encounter none at all.

HOW KAVA CAN HELP A traditional "remedy" for menopause is hormone replacement therapy. This optional treatment uses synthetic hormones to elevate progesterone and oestrogen to their premenopausal levels. Kava is helpful regardless of whether one undergoes or forgoes hormone replacement therapy. Several studies have found kava successful in treating the emotional symptoms that sometimes accompany the condition; the herb's mood-improving and sedating powers help elevate a depressed mood, alleviate irritability and nervousness, and promote normal sleep. Furthermore, kava is also a gentle diuretic and acts to flush retained water from the body, thus treating general puffiness and localized swelling.

DOSAGES Take 250mg extract three times daily, or ½ teaspoon of tincture three times a day.

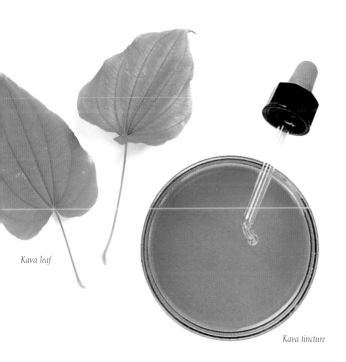

Kava leaf

Kava tincture

ADJUSTMENT DISORDER

SYMPTOMS This is also called situational or reactive depression, because it occurs in reaction to a traumatic or stressful event that has transpired within the preceding three months. Symptoms can include decreased self-esteem, grief, helplessness, impaired daily functioning, irritability, sense of doom, and social withdrawal. Adjustment disorder generally disappears on its own within six months, although a small number of cases worsen into a major depressive disorder.

HOW KAVA CAN HELP The kavalactones found in kava affect the limbic system, a part of the brain that helps regulate mood and is the principal seat of the emotions.

Note: *Consider seeing a trained councillor who can help speed your healing.*

DOSAGES Take 250mg extract three times daily, or ½ teaspoon of tincture three times daily. You should begin seeing mild changes within a couple of days and more dramatic improvement after a week. Discontinue when mood is stabilized.

· THE KAVA CEREMONY ·

Throughout the Pacific islands kava is made into a beverage, which stars in several different celebrational and welcoming ceremonies. Once upon a time, kava drinks were prepared by young, unmarried women, who cut kava root into pieces, chewed each piece into a pulp, then spat the pulp into a container. The liquid from several coconuts was poured over the masticated root and the whole mixture allowed to sit for up to a day. Right before serving, the concoction was strained and served in coconut bowls.

In 1777 a naturalist named Georg Forster accompanied James Cook on the latter's second Pacific voyage. After watching kava beverages being made and drunk, Forster had this to say: "They swallow this nauseous stuff as fast as possible; and some old topers value themselves on being able to empty a great number of bowls."

Kava drinks continued being made and enjoyed after Europeans settled the region. However, the newcomers encouraged islanders to use more sanitary methods of preparation, and grating or grinding the root eventually replaced chewing it.

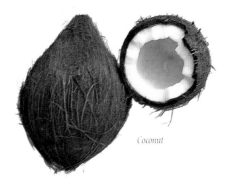

Coconut

ANXIETY DISORDER

SYMPTOMS Also called generalized anxiety disorder, this condition features persistent anxiety for at least one month. Anxiety disorder may have a discernible catalyst (such as fear of redundancy), but often there is no triggering event. Symptoms include apprehension, difficulty concentrating, dizziness, dry mouth, gastrointestinal distress, headaches, unusually heavy perspiration, impatience, inability to relax, insomnia, irritability, muscle aches, muscle tension, rapid heartbeat, restlessness, shortness of breath, night-time teeth grinding, and tension. Individuals may also experience random attacks of terror known as panic attacks.

HOW KAVA CAN HELP Kava's traditional use in the Pacific islands is as an anti-anxiety medication. German doctors also prescribe kava to combat anxiety. It isn't known exactly how kava works, although the herb has a sedative effect on the central nervous system and is also known to target the limbic system, which controls moods.

Note: *Consider seeing a trained councillor who can help speed your healing.*

DOSAGES Take 250mg extract three times daily; or ½ teaspoon of tincture three times daily. You should begin seeing mild changes within a couple of days and more dramatic improvement after a week. Discontinue when mood has stabilized.

· KAVA VS. PRESCRIBED ·
ANTI-ANXIETY MEDICATIONS

In certain parts of Europe kava is regularly used to treat anxiety disorder, stress, and temporary nervousness. But doctors are still more likely to prescribe anti-anxiety medications, in particular benzodiazapenes, which work by mimicking the actions of gamma-amino-butyric acid. Known as GABA, this neurotransmitter (brain chemical) has a soothing effect on the body. Unfortunately, while benzodiazapenes diminish anxiousness, their effectiveness comes with side-effects, most notably appetite change, blurred vision, diarrhoea, dizziness, dry mouth, ringing in the ears, slowed mental reactions, slowed physical reactions, and temporary short-term memory impairment.

A European study comparing 19 people on various anti-anxiety medications (including Xanax and Valium) to 19 people taking kava found both groups reported decreased anxiety after four weeks. However, all individuals on synthetic anti-anxiety medications reported at least one of the side effects listed above, while the kava takers experienced no side effects.

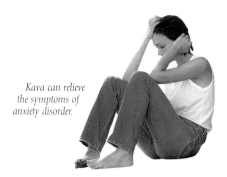

Kava can relieve the symptoms of anxiety disorder.

DEPRESSION

SYMPTOMS The condition often begins with no apparent trigger, though it can also develop from adjustment disorder. Symptoms can include change in appetite, decreased self-esteem, grief, helplessness, impaired daily functioning, irritability, loss of interest in previously enjoyable activities, inappropriate guilt, lethargy, malaise, neglect of physical appearance, self-reproach, sense of doom, sleep disturbances, slowed physical and mental responses, social withdrawal, and thoughts of suicide.

HOW KAVA CAN HELP While St John's wort is the world's most-prescribed herbal antidepressant, kava ranks just below it. Again the effect may be largely via the limbic system, a part of the brain that helps regulate moods and controls emotions.

Note: *While mild depression can be successfully treated with kava alone, the illness responds best to a combination of therapy and kava. Moderate depression responds best to a combination of the two.*

DOSAGES Take 250mg extract three times daily, or ½ teaspoon of tincture three times daily. You should begin seeing mild changes within a couple of days and more dramatic improvement after a week. Discontinue when mood has stabilized.

· TOO MUCH OF A GOOD THING ·

As with any herb, there is such a thing as too much kava.
In kava's case, too much is 310–440gm (310,000–440,000mgs)
consumed weekly for two to three months. Though doses this
high are rare, they are sometimes seen in the South Pacific
islands. The consequences of this much kava? A condition
known as kawaism, or kawa dermopathy, which is
characterized by reddened eyes, scaly skin, and a yellowish
discolouration of hair, nails, skin, and the whites of the eyes.
(This discolouration is attributed to two of the plant's yellow
pigments.) Fortunately, side effects disappear when kava
consumption is reduced or stopped.

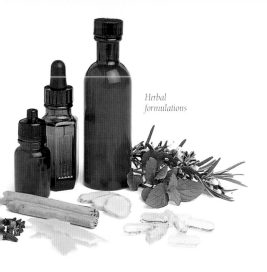

*Herbal
formulations*

INSOMNIA

SYMPTOMS Insomnia is the medical name for inadequate sleep that occurs for at least one week. Among the causes are noisy environment, high caffeine or alcohol intake, an existing illness, and stress. Yet regardless of what causes insomnia, the result is the same: daytime tiredness. Symptoms can include difficulty falling asleep, not sleeping deeply enough, waking during the night and not being able to fall back to sleep, waking too early in the morning, and waking and falling back to sleep sporadically throughout the night.

HOW KAVA CAN HELP One of kava's traditional uses is as a sedative, and there is evidence that kava increases deep sleep. Kava is thought to benefit insomniacs indirectly through beneficially affecting emotional well being, as well as having a sedative effect on the central nervous system.

DOSAGES Take 500mg extract one hour before retiring. For less severe sleep problems, drinking 1 or 2 cups of kava tea or taking a warm bath with 1 teaspoon of kava tincture, or ½ teaspoon of essential oil may do the trick.

· HELP FOR INSOMNIACS ·

◆ Don't drink caffeinated drinks after 2pm or 3pm. Caffeine can upset your body's natural time clock.

◆ Don't exercise within four hours of going to bed. Vigorous physical activity can temporarily energize the body, making sleep difficult.

◆ Trade adrenaline-pumping television shows for a relaxing book.

◆ Because the human body prefers a faithfully kept schedule, try to retire at the same time each night.

◆ Lower the lights. Some sleep experts believe bright lights during the evening can hamper sleep. How? By tricking your body's internal time clock into thinking it is earlier in the day.

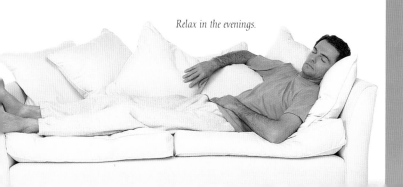

Relax in the evenings.

STRESS

SYMPTOMS Whether caused by increased demands at work, money worries, relationship woes, or something else entirely, stress prompts the body to release what are called stress hormones, such as epinephrine and cortisol. These hormones help increase blood flow to the muscles and prepare the body for a short period of extreme exertion. However, in times of ongoing anxiety, high levels of these hormones hang around in the body, causing changes in appetite, gastrointestinal upset, headaches, impaired concentration, irritability, muscle tension, sleeplessness, and night-time teeth grinding.

HOW KAVA CAN HELP For centuries Pacific islanders have used kava to reduce stress. Indeed, several German studies have shown that kava greatly diminishes or alleviates symptoms of stress. The effect is thought to be through kava's effect on the central nervous system and limbic system, which stabilizes moods and controls emotions.

DOSAGES Take 250mg extract three times daily. A relaxing kava bath is also helpful. To a warm bath, add one teaspoon of kava tincture, or ½ teaspoon of essential oil.

· KAVA VS. ALCOHOL ·

Many researchers have likened kava's "social" effects to those of alcohol. Indeed, there does seem to be a resemblance. Both loosen the tongue, diminish shyness, and dampen inhibitions. But the similarities end there. Unlike alcohol, kava is not intoxicating or physically addictive, and those who use it do not develop a tolerance that forces them to use more over time to reap the benefits. When taken in 250mg doses or lower, kava does not affect motor skills, and unlike alcohol, the herb seems to slightly improve mental functioning. Even in very high doses kava is not as physically debilitating as alcohol. In one study, a group of young adults were given six pints of kava beverage over a two-hour period – an enormous amount. Though the students acted sleepy and developed bloodshot eyes, they had no trouble walking a straight line and easily ran up staircases two steps at a time. And unlike alcohol, kava (even in high doses) does not produce a "hangover" the next day.

BACK PAIN

SYMPTOMS Back pain is usually caused by pulled, strained, or weak muscles. A sprain occurs when a violent twist of stretch causes the joint to move outside its normal range of movement, injuring the muscles or ligaments that connect the bones.

HOW KAVA CAN HELP Kava acts on contracted muscles, relaxing them and easing pain. If it is applied topically (as an essential oil, for example) it also has a mild anaesthetic effect. Finally, kava's sedative effect helps reduce the anxiousness that often accompanies muscle or joint pain.

DOSAGES Gently massage the area up to three times a day with a kava essential oil suitably diluted in a carrier essential oil. To further reduce pain, take 250mg extract three times daily, or ½ tsp tincture three times daily.

SPRAINED MUSCLES

SYMPTOMS A sprain occurs when a violent twist or stretch causes the joint to move outside its normal range of movement, injuring the muscles and/or ligaments that connect the bones. The result is rapid swelling in the injured area, impaired joint function, pain, and tenderness.

HOW KAVA CAN HELP Kava acts on damaged muscles, relaxing them and easing pain. If it is applied topically (as an essential oil, for example) it also has a mild anaesthetic effect. Finally, kava's sedative effect helps reduce the anxiousness that often accompanies muscle or joint pain.

DOSAGES Apply a kava poultice or fomentation to the affected area up to three times daily until the area heals. Or gently massage the area up to three times a day with a kava essential oil suitably diluted in a carrier essential oil. To further reduce pain, take 250mg extract three times daily, or ½ tsp tincture three times daily. Another option is a relaxing kava bath: add ½ teaspoon of essential oil, or one teaspoon of tincture to a warm bath.

STROKE

SYMPTOMS A stroke is a cerebrovascular condition characterized by a blockage of blood to any given part of the brain. A stroke leaves a portion of the brain temporarily without oxygen-rich blood, thus killing the brain tissue and leaving a stroke survivor with diminished brain function. There are several risk factors for strokes, including coronary artery disease, genetics, high blood pressure, high cholesterol diet, and smoking. A stroke can occur over a few seconds, minutes, or even hours, and can be moderate, severe, or fatal. Symptoms may include deterioration in sensation, speech, or vision over a period of hours or minutes; headache; uncoordination; loss of consciousness; and sudden weakness or paralysis in an arm and/or a leg.

HOW KAVA CAN HELP Researchers don't yet know how kava affects the brain, only that it does to do so. One theory is that it may somehow help to protect the brain tissues, acting as a "neuroprotective" agent.

DOSAGES As a preventative, take 250mg extract three times daily, or ½ teaspoon of tincture three times daily. Kava can also be taken in the same dosages after a first stroke to help prevent a second stroke.

· STROKE FACTS ·

◆ Approximately 300,000 Americans suffer a stroke each year; a quarter of these individuals die and half have long-term disabilities.

◆ Strokes are the third leading cause of death in developed countries.

◆ The risk of having a stroke doubles each decade after age 35.

◆ Around 100,000 people in England and Wales have a first stroke each year – one every five minutes.

◆ Anyone can have a stroke, including babies and children, but the vast majority – nine out of 10 – affect people over 55.

◆ Seventy per cent of all strokes occur in people with high blood pressure.

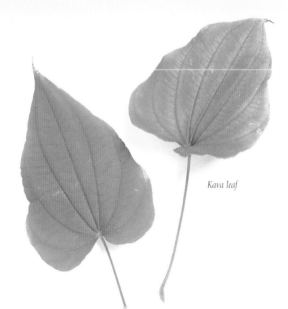

Kava leaf

TENSION HEADACHE

SYMPTOMS Tension headaches are also known as muscle-contraction headaches because they occur when the cranial and/or cervical muscles covering the skull contract. The resulting pain is vice-like, located at the scalp, temples, or back of the neck, and can be moderate to intense. The most common cause of head pain, tension headaches can be caused by anxiety, depression, poor posture, strain, stress, or working in awkward positions.

HOW KAVA CAN HELP Kava is traditionally used in the Pacific islands to treat headaches. The herb works in two ways: the kavalactones in kava relax tight, constricted muscles, thus loosening the grip of cranial or cervical muscles, and the herb's analgesic power deadens pain.

DOSAGES At the first sign of symptoms, enjoy 1 or or 2 cups of kava tea. For stronger relief, take up to three doses of 250mg extract within a 24-hour period, or three ½-teaspoon doses of tincture within a 24-hour period.

· MIGRAINES ·

A migraine is quite different from a tension headache; it differs in several respects.

MIGRAINE:

◆ Location of pain on one side of head/both sides of head.

◆ Duration of pain: 4–72 hours.

◆ Symptoms can include nausea, sensitivity to light, sound, and odours.

◆ Possibility of redness of eyes, or tears, and a stuffy and runny nose.

TENSION-TYPE:

◆ Location of pain on both sides of head.

◆ Duration of pain: 2 hours to several days.

If you think you might suffer from migraines seek medical advice, as migraines often need to be treated in a different way from ordinary tension headaches.

DO-IT-YOURSELF REMEDIES

CAPSULE You can make your own herbal supplements by purchasing animal or vegetable gelatin capsules at your local health food store and packing each capsule with 250mg extract powdered kava leaves.

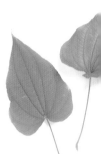

DECOCTION Because kava root is less permeable than the aerial parts of the plant, simmering the root in boiling water helps extract a greater percentage of its medicinal constituents. To make a decoction, place 25g of chopped dried root or 75g chopped fresh root in a nonreactive saucepan. Cover with 750ml cold water, place a lid on the saucepan, and boil until the liquid reduces to 500ml. Strain the liquid and use warm or allow to cool.

DRYING Wash, thoroughly dry, and chop fresh kava root into small pieces. Lay the chopped herb on trays in a dry, well-ventilated, shaded area of your home, or place in an oven on a very low temperature, making sure air is continually circulating around the herbs, or use a dehydrator. Drying will take between seven and 14 days. When drying herbs either in a warm room or in an oven, the temperature should be kept between 20°-30°C (70°-90°F). Store the dried root in a dark, airtight, nonporous container.

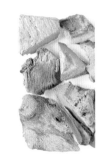

FOMENTATION Fomentations are essentially gauze or surgical bandages soaked in freshly made herbal tea. The hot cloth is then laid directly on a sprained or strained muscle.

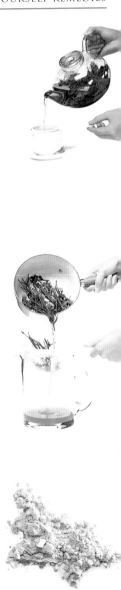

INFUSED OIL Infused oils boast the fat-soluble active principles of whatever medicinal plant or herb has been used to make them. To make kava oil, place 200g of dried kava root in a nonreactive saucepan and cover with 500ml almond or olive oil. Simmer over a very low heat for three hours. Allow mixture to cool. Strain the oil and store in a dark, airtight container for up to two years. Infused oil can be ingested or used externally.

LIQUID EXTRACT Also known as extract. To make kava extract, macerate 100-200g of dried kava root, or 300-500g of fresh root. Place the herb in a jar and pour in 335ml vodka (40% alcohol by volume) and 165ml water. Screw the lid on the jar and store in a dark area for four to eight weeks. Shake the mixture daily. When ready, strain the mixture, pressing all remaining liquid from the ginkgo leaves. Place liquid in a nonreactive saucepan and simmer over medium heat for 20-40 minutes until the liquid has been reduced by a third. This process burns off the alcohol, leaving the medicinal liquid behind. Allow the liquid to cool and decant into several dropper bottles or a clean glass bottle. Will keep up to two years. Shake before using.

OINTMENT Also called a salve, herbal ointment is easy to make at home. To create your own kava ointment, mix 1 to 2 parts beeswax or soft paraffin wax, 7 parts cocoa butter, and 3 parts dried, powdered kava root in a nonreactive saucepan. Cook the mixture for one to two hours on a low setting. Leave to cool, package in an airtight container, and apply up to three times a day when required.

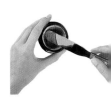

POULTICE Fresh herbs can be applied directly to the skin when fashioned into a poultice. To make a kava poultice, chop the fresh or dried root. Boil in a small amount of water for five minutes (or use a microwave). Squeeze out any excess liquid from the boiled herb (reserve liquid). Lay the kava directly on to the skin and cover with a warm moist towel. Leave in place for up to 30 minutes. The reserved liquid can be rewarmed.

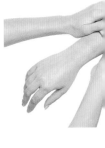

SYRUP Kava has a bitter taste that may not be palatable to some individuals. Syrup delivers the herb's medicinal benefits in an easy-to-swallow (and throat-soothing) base. To make, mix 7 parts of kava tea or decoction in a nonreactive saucepan with 10 parts sugar. Cook the mixture over a low heat until it has formed a thick, syrupy consistency.

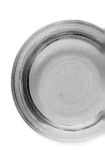

TEA Also known as an infusion, tea is an easy and common way to ingest an herb. To make kava tea, steep 1 teaspoon of dried root or 1 tablespoon fresh leaves for five minutes in a cup of boiling water. You may want to add fructose, sugar, or honey to sweeten the infusion.

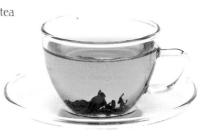

TINCTURES Though they are not as potent as liquid extracts, tinctures are minimally processed, making them a favourite remedy among herbalists. To make your own kava tincture, place 100-200g of dried kava root or 300-500g of fresh kava root in a large jar and cover with 500ml vodka (40% alcohol by volume). Place the lid on the jar and store in a dark area for four to six weeks. Shake the bottle daily. When ready to use strain the mixture, pressing all remaining liquid from the leaves. Decant into several dropper bottles or a clean glass bottle. Will keep for up to a year. Shake before using.

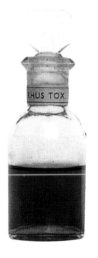

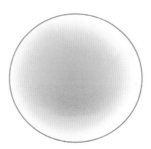

ALTERNATIVE HEALTH STRATEGIES

Herbs, vitamins, and minerals all contribute to good health. However, creating a sense of general well-being involves more than simply taking supplements. Health has to do with a quality of life that can often be aggravated by causes of harmful stress. Listed below are some additional ways to help keep yourself well.

IMPROVE YOUR EATING HABITS

Listed below are the five main eating strategies people follow; consider finding the healthiest one that suits your lifestyle.

- Omnivore
- Semi-vegetarian
- Macrobiotic
- Vegan
- Vegetarian

Legumes

GET MORE EXERCISE

Whether it's walking or weightlifting, any type of exercise can help you feel better. Try any of these types:

- Stretching
- Aerobics
- Resistance training

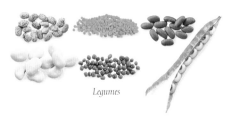

Exercise by walking as much as possible.

SIMPLE WAYS TO EASE STRESS

In addition to exercise and healthy eating, here are some more techniques – old and new – for easing stress and increasing relaxation.

◆ Get enough sleep
◆ Take time to relax
◆ Give up junk food
◆ Adopt a pet
◆ Surround yourself with supportive people
◆ Limit your exposure to chemicals
◆ Enjoy yourself

‣ ONE-MINUTE STRESS REDUCER ‣

Deep breathing can be done anywhere and anytime you need to calm and centre yourself:

1 Inhale deeply through your nose.
2 Hold your breath for up to three seconds, then exhale your breath through your mouth.
3 Continue as needed.

Deep breathing draws a person's attention away from a given stress and refocuses it on his or her breathing. This type of breathing is not only comforting (thanks to its rhythmic quality), but also has been shown to lower rapid pulse and shallow respiration – two temporary symptoms of stress.

GET MOVING

Ask medical experts to name one stay-young strategy and there's a good chance that "exercise" will be the answer. And with good reason. Exercise, whether a gentle walk around the block or a full-tilt weight lifting session, strengthens the heart, lowers the body's resting heart rate, builds muscles, boosts circulation to the body and the brain, revs up the metabolism and burns calories. All of which can keep a person looking and feeling his or her best. For it to be effective, exercise several times a week. Aim for at least three sessions. For optimum health, try a combination of aerobic exercise and strength training. And don't forget to stretch before and after each workout!

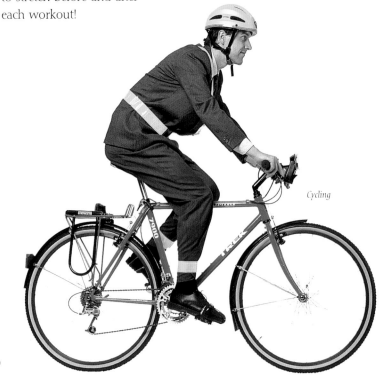

Cycling

STRETCHING

WHAT IT IS Any movement that stretches muscles. Examples include bending at the waist and touching the toes, sitting with legs outstretched in front of you, and rolling your neck. Stretch for eight to twelve minutes before every workout and again after you exercise.

WHY IT'S IMPORTANT Muscles act like springs. If a muscle is short and tight, it loses the ability to absorb shock. The less shock a muscle can absorb, the more strain there is on the joints. Thus, stretching maintains flexibility, which in turn prevents injuries. Because we often lose our regular range of motion with age, stretching is especially important for older adults to prevent sprains, strains and falls.

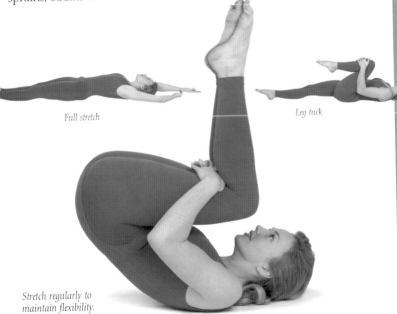

Full stretch

Leg tuck

Stretch regularly to maintain flexibility.

AEROBICS

WHAT IT IS Any activity that uses large muscle groups, is maintained continuously for 15 minutes or more, and is rhythmic in nature. Examples include aerobic dance, jogging, skating and walking. Ideally, you should aim for three to six aerobic workouts per week.

WHY IT'S IMPORTANT Aerobic exercise trains the heart, lungs, and cardiovascular system to process and deliver oxygen more quickly and efficiently to every part of the body. As the heart muscle becomes stronger and more efficient, a larger amount of blood can be pumped with each stroke. Fewer strokes are then required to rapidly transport oxygen to all parts of the body.

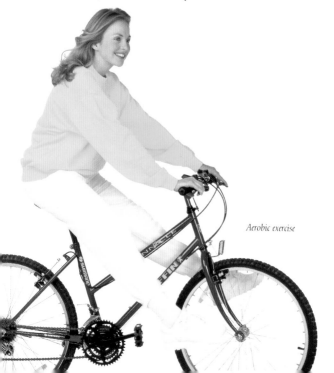

Aerobic exercise

RESISTANCE TRAINING

WHAT IT IS Any activity that improves the condition of your muscles by making repeated movements against a force. Examples include lifting large or small weights, sit-ups, stair-stepping, and isometrics.

WHY IT'S IMPORTANT Resistance training makes it easier to move heavy loads, whether they require carrying, pushing, pulling, or lifting, as well as participating in sports that require strength. The exercises are of various kinds. Some require changing the length of the muscle while maintaining the level of tension, others involve using special equipment to vary the tension in the muscles, and some entail contracting a muscle while maintaining its length.

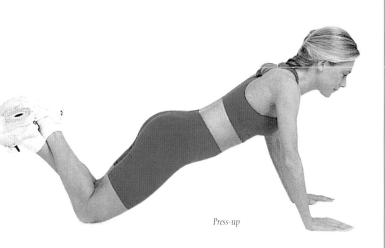

Press-up

POPULAR EATING STRATEGIES

EATING SMART

A balanced diet is the foundation of good health. For proof, just read the numerous medical studies that link healthy eating with disease prevention and disease reversal. These same studies connect high fat intake, high sodium consumption, and diets with too much protein to numerous illnesses, including cancer, cardiovascular diseases, diverticular diseases, hypertension, and heart disease. But what exactly is a balanced diet? Generally speaking, it is a diet comprised of carbohydrates, dietary fibre, fat, protein, water, 13 vitamins and 20 minerals. More specifically, it is a diet built around a wide variety of fruits, legumes, whole grains, and vegetables. Alcohol, animal protein, high-fat foods, high-sodium foods, highly-sugared foods, fizzy drinks, and processed foods are consumed sparingly.

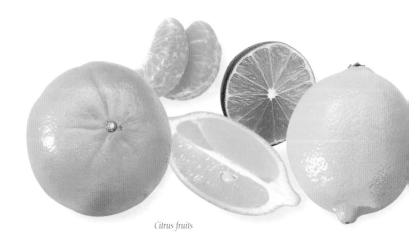

Citrus fruits

OMNIVOROUS

ON THE MENU Plant-based foods, dairy products, eggs, fish, seafood, red meats, organ meats, poultry.

FOODS THAT ARE AVOIDED None. Everything is fair game.

HOW HEALTHY IS IT? It depends. Someone who eats eggs, poultry, or meat every day, chooses refined snacks over whole foods, and gets only one or two daily servings of fruits and vegetables will not be as healthy as a person who limits meat (the general dietary term for any "flesh foods", including poultry and fish) to two or three times a week, chooses water over soft drinks, and gets the recommended five or more daily servings of fruits and vegetables. Complaints about traditional omnivorous diets revolve around the diet's high levels of cholesterol and saturated fat (found in animal-based foods), which increase the risk of cancer, diabetes, heart disease, and obesity. However, an omnivorous diet can be healthful one provided thoughtful choices are made. To keep cholesterol and saturated fat to a minimum and nutrients to a maximum, eat five or more daily servings of fruits and vegetables, choose whole grains over refined grains, enjoy daily legume or soyfood protein sources, and limit the use of animal foods.

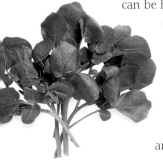

Watercress

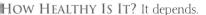

Egg

Semi-vegetarian

On The Menu Plant-based foods, dairy products, eggs, fish, seafood.

Foods That Are Avoided Red meats, organ meats, poultry.

How Healthy Is It? Like an omnivorous diet, a semi-vegetarian diet is as healthy as a person makes it. Individuals who eat high-fat and highly processed foods fail to get the recommended daily number of vegetables and fruits, and eschew whole grains for processed grains will not enjoy optimum health. That said, individuals who are conscientious about eating a balanced, varied diet, and who limit fish and seafood intake to two or three times per week, can expect a lower risk of heart disease. Since many oily fish contain omega-3 fatty acids, eating them in moderation has been found to help lower blood cholesterol. Be aware, however, that oily saltwater fish such as shark, swordfish and tuna have been found to carry mercury in their tissues; many health authorities recommend eating these varieties no more than once or twice a week. Also, due to overfishing, many fish species are now threatened, including bluefin tuna, Pacific perch, Chilean sea bass, Chinook salmon, and swordfish.

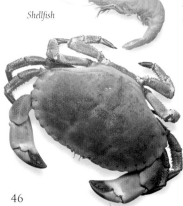

Shellfish

MACROBIOTIC

ON THE MENU Plant-based foods, fish, very limited amounts of salt.

FOODS THAT ARE AVOIDED Dairy products, eggs, foods with artificial ingredients, hot spices, mass-produced foods, organ meats, peppers, potatoes, poultry, red meats, shellfish, warm drinks, and refined foods.

HOW HEALTHY IS IT? Macrobiotics is based on a system created in the early 1900s by Japanese philosopher George Ohsawa. The diet consists of 50 per cent whole grains, 20-30 per cent vegetables, and 5-10 per cent beans, sea vegetables, and soy foods. The remainder of the diet is composed of white-meat fish, fruits, and nuts. The diet's low amounts of saturated fat, absence of processed foods, and emphasis on high-fibre foods such as whole grains and vegetables, may promote cardiovascular health. Because soy and sea vegetables contain cancer-fighting compounds, a macrobiotic diet is often recommended to help treat cancer. However, critics worry that the diet's limited variety of food can leave followers lacking in certain vitamins and important cancer-fighting phytonutrients.

Leafy green vegetables

VEGAN

ON THE MENU Plant-based foods.

FOODS THAT ARE AVOIDED Dairy, eggs, fish, seafood, red meats, organ meats, poultry. Also avoided are foods made by animals or processed with animal parts, such as gelatin, honey, marshmallows made with animal gelatin, white sugar processed with bone char.

HOW HEALTHY IS IT? A vegan (pronounced VEE-gun) diet can be extremely healthful. Like the vegetarian diet, a vegan diet has been shown by numerous studies to lower blood pressure and prevent heart disease. In addition, the high fibre intake cuts the risk of diverticular disease and colon cancer. Yet because vegans do not eat dairy products or eggs, they must be more conscientious than vegetarians about eating plant foods with vitamin B12 and vitamin D or taking supplements of these nutrients.

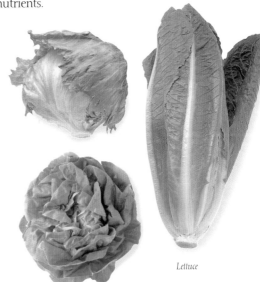

Lettuce

VEGETARIAN

ON THE MENU Plant-based foods, dairy, eggs.

FOODS THAT ARE AVOIDED Fish, gelatin, seafood, red meats, organ meats, poultry.

HOW HEALTHY IS IT? A vegetarian diet can be very healthy when done right. Fortunately, this isn't hard. Dietary science has debunked theories of "protein combining" popular in the 1960s and 1970s, leaving today's vegetarians to worry only about eating a wide variety of whole foods including beans, fruits, grains, low-fat dairy products, nuts, soy foods, and vegetables. A varied daily diet insures enough protein, calcium, and other nutrients for vegetarians of all ages, including children, pregnant individuals, and the elderly. A well-chosen vegetarian eating plan has been shown by numerous studies to lower blood pressure, decrease the risk of breast cancer, and prevent heart disease. In addition, the diet's high fibre levels cut the risk of diverticular disease and colon cancer.

Sweet potato

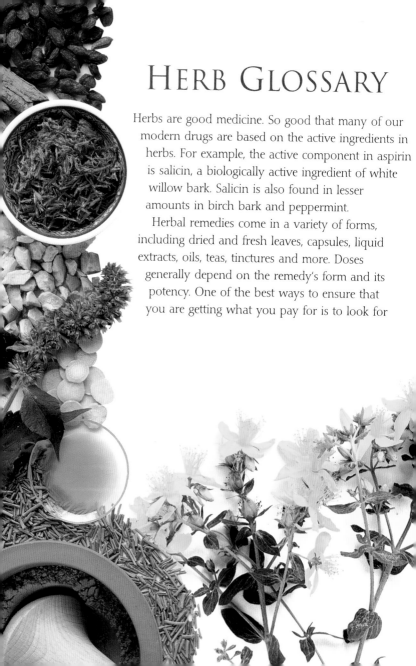

HERB GLOSSARY

Herbs are good medicine. So good that many of our modern drugs are based on the active ingredients in herbs. For example, the active component in aspirin is salicin, a biologically active ingredient of white willow bark. Salicin is also found in lesser amounts in birch bark and peppermint.

Herbal remedies come in a variety of forms, including dried and fresh leaves, capsules, liquid extracts, oils, teas, tinctures and more. Doses generally depend on the remedy's form and its potency. One of the best ways to ensure that you are getting what you pay for is to look for a product with a standardized extract. This guarantees that the remedy will contain the stated percentage of the herb's active ingredient.

One last note: herbal remedies have an ancient track record for safety. However, they can cause harm when used incorrectly or by individuals with contraindications. If you are unsure of whether an herb is for you, please contact your doctor or a naturopathic doctor.

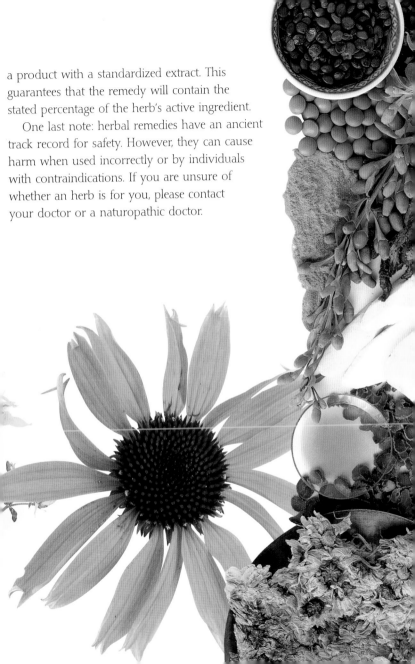

ACHILLEA MILLEFOLIUM
Yarrow

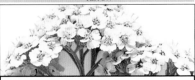

Properties Antibacterial, anti-inflammatory, antispasmodic, blood coagulator, bile stimulating, immune-system stimulant, promotes sweating, sedative.

Target Ailments Anxiety, colds and flu, cystitis, digestive disorders, menstrual cramps, minor wounds, nosebleeds, poor circulation, skin rashes.

Available Forms Dried herb, capsule, liquid extract, oil, tea, tincture.

Possible Side Effects Diarrhoea, skin rash.

Precautions Yarrow is related to ragweed and can cause an allergic reaction in individuals with ragweed allergies. Do not take if pregnant; it can induce miscarriage.

ALLIUM SATIVUM
Garlic

Properties Antibacterial, anticoagulant, antifungal, anti-inflammatory, antiviral, cholesterol reducer, digestive aid, immune-system stimulant, worm-fighting.

Target Ailments Arteriosclerosis, arthritis, bladder infections, colds, digestive upset, flu, heart conditions, high blood pressure, high blood cholesterol, viral infections.

Available Forms Capsule, fresh cloves, liquid extract, oil, tincture.

Possible Side Effects Can cause upset stomach.

Precautions While garlic is safe taken in culinary doses, individuals on anticoagulant medications should consult their doctor before supplementing their diet with garlic.

ASTRAGALUS SPP.
Astragalus

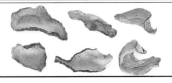

Properties Antibacterial, anti-inflammatory, antioxidant, antiviral, diuretic, immune-system stimulant.

Target Ailments Cancer, colds, appetite loss, diarrhoea, fatigue, flu, heart conditions, HIV, viral infections.

Available Forms Capsule, dried herb, fresh herb, liquid extract, tea, tincture.

Possible Side Effects None expected.

Precautions Astragalus should be used as a companion therapy to – not a replacement for – traditional cancer and HIV therapies.

CALENDULA OFFICINALIS
Calendula

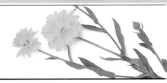

Properties Antibacterial, anti-inflammatory, antiseptic, antispasmodic, promotes sweating, sedative.

Target Ailments Burns, cuts, fungal infection, gallbladder conditions, hepatitis, indigestion, irregular menstruation, insect bites, menstrual cramps, mouth sores, skin rashes, ulcers, wounds.

Available Forms Capsule, dried herb, fresh herb, liquid extract, lotion, oil, ointment, tincture.

Possible Side Effects None expected.

Precautions Calendula is related to ragweed. Individuals allergic to ragweed should consult a doctor before using calendula.

ALOE VERA
Aloe

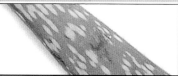

Properties Analgesic, antibacterial, antifungal, anti-inflammatory, anti-itch, antiseptic, circulatory stimulant, digestive aid, immune-system stimulant, laxative.

Target Ailments Acne, bruises, burns, constipation, cuts, insect bites, digestive disorders, rashes, ulcers, wounds.

Available Forms Capsule, fresh leaves, gel, juice, liquid extract.

Possible Side Effects When taken internally, aloe can cause severe cramping in some individuals.

Precautions Pregnant women should not ingest aloe; It can stimulate uterine contractions.

ANGELICA POLYMORPHA
Dong Quai

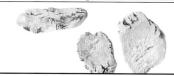

Properties Antiallergenic, antispasmodic, diuretic, mild laxative, muscle relaxant, vasodilator.

Target Ailments Abscesses, blurred vision, heart palpitations, irregular menstruation, light-headedness, menstrual pain, pallor, poor circulation.

Available Forms Capsule, dried herb, liquid extract, tincture.

Possible Side Effects Can cause photosensitivity in some individuals.

Precautions Dong quai has abortive abilities; Do not take while pregnant.

CHAMAEMELUM NOBILE
Chamomile

Properties Antibacterial, anti-inflammatory, antiseptic, antispasmodic, carminative, digestive aid, fever reducer, sedative.

Target Ailments Gingivitis, haemorrhoids, insomnia, indigestion, intestinal gas, menstrual cramps, nausea, nervousness, stomachaches, sunburns, tension, ulcers, varicose veins.

Available Forms Capsule, dried herb, fresh herb, liquid extract, lotion, oil, tea, tincture.

Possible Side Effects None expected.

Precautions Because chamomile is related to ragweed, individuals with ragweed allergies should consult a doctor before using chamomile.

DIOSCOREA VILLOSA
Wild Yam

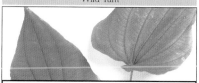

Properties Analgesic, anti-inflammatory, antispasmodic, expectorant, muscle relaxant, promotes sweating.

Target Ailments Menopause, menstrual cramps, morning sickness, nausea, rheumatoid arthritis, urinary tract infections.

Available Forms Capsule, cream, dried root, liquid extract, oil, powder, tincture.

Possible Side Effects Can cause vomiting in large doses.

Precautions Individuals who are suffering from a hormone-sensitive cancer, such as breast or uterine cancer, should avoid wild yam. Some experts believe that the herb can encourage the growth of cancer cells.

ECHINACEA PURPUREA
Echinacea

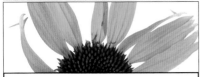

Properties Antiallergenic, antibacterial, antiseptic, antimicrobial, antiviral, carminative, lymphatic tonic.

Target Ailments Abscesses, acne, bladder infections, blood poisoning, burns, colds, eczema, food poisoning, flu, insect bites, kidney infections, mononucleosis, respiratory infections, sore throats.

Available Forms Capsule, dried herb, liquid extract, tea, tincture.

Possible Side Effects High doses can cause dizziness and nausea.

Precautions Do not take echinacea for more than four weeks in a row.

GINKGO BILOBA
Ginkgo

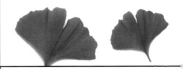

Properties Antibacterial, anti-inflammatory, antioxidant, circulatory stimulant, vasodilator.

Target Ailments Clotting disorders, dementia, depression, headaches, hearing loss, Raynaud's syndrome, tinnitus, vascular diseases, vertigo.

Available Forms Capsule, dry herb, liquid extract, tincture, tea.

Possible Side Effects Diarrhoea, irritability, nausea, restlessness.

Precautions Do not use ginkgo biloba if you have a blood-clotting disorder like haemophilia or are taking anticoagulant medications.

LAVANDULA SPP.
Lavender

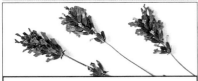

Properties Antibacterial, antidepressant, antiseptic, antispasmodic, carminative, circulatory stimulant, digestive aid, diuretic, sedative.

Target Ailments Anxiety, depression, headache, insomnia, intestinal gas, nausea, tension.

Available Forms Capsule, dried herb, fresh herb, oil, tincture.

Possible Side Effects Lavender products can cause skin irritation in sensitive individuals.

Precautions Lavender oil is poisonous when ingested internally.

MENTHA PIPERITA
Peppermint

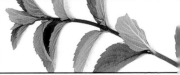

Properties Antacid, antibacterial, antidepressant, antispasmodic, carminatve, expectorant, muscle relaxant, promotes sweating.

Target Ailments Anxiety, colds, fever, flu, insomnia, intestinal gas, itching, migraines, morning sickness, motion sickness, nausea.

Available Forms Capsule, dried herb, fresh herb, lozenge, oil, ointment, tea, tincture.

Possible Side Effects When applied externally peppermint products can cause skin reactions in sensitive individuals.

Precautions If you have a hiatal hernia, talk to your doctor before using peppermint products externally or internally; the oil in the plant can exacerbate symptoms.

HYDRASTIS CANADENSIS
Goldenseal

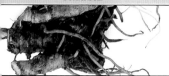

Properties Antacid, antibacterial, antifungal, anti-inflammatory, antiseptic, astringent, digestive aid, stimulant.

Target Ailments Canker sores, contact dermatitis, diarrhoea, eczema, food poisoning. **Available Forms** Capsule, dry herb, liquid extract, tea, tincture.

Possible Side Effects In high doses, goldenseal can cause diarrhoea and nausea and can irritate the skin, mouth and throat.

Precautions Because of its high cost, many manufacturers adulterate preparations with less costly herbs, such as barberry, yellow dock or bloodroot, some of which can cause unwanted reactions when taken in high doses.

HYPERICUM PERFORATUM
St John's wort

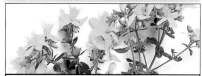

Properties Analgesic, antibacterial, anti-depressant, anti-inflammatory, antiviral, astringent.

Target Ailments Attention deficit disorder, anxiety, bacterial infections, burns, carpal tunnel syndrome, depression. menopause.

Available Forms Capsule, dried herb, liquid extract, oil, ointment, tea, tincture.

Possible Side Effects Gastrointestinal upset, headaches, photosensitivity, stiff neck.

Precautions Avoid foods containing the amino acid tyramine when taking St John's wort; the interaction of the two can cause an increase in blood pressure. Foods with tyramine include beer, coffee, wine, chocolate and fava beans.

PENAX SPP.
Ginseng

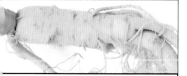

Properties Antibacterial, antidepressant, immune-system stimulant, stimulant.

Target Ailments Colds, depression, fatigue, impaired immune system, respiratory conditions, stress.

Available Forms Capsule, dried root, fresh root, liquid extract, tincture, tea.

Possible Side Effects Large doses of ginseng can cause breast soreness, headaches or skin rashes in some individuals.

Precautions Ginseng can aggravate existing heart palpitations or high blood pressure.

PETROSELINUM CRISPUM
Parsley

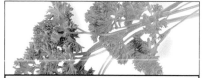

Properties Antiseptic, antispasmodic, digestive aid, diuretic, laxative, muscle relaxant.

Target Ailments Colds, congestion, fever, flu, indigestion, irregular menstruation, premenstrual syndrome, stimulating the production of breast milk, stomachaches.

Available Forms Capsule, dried herb, fresh herb, liquid extract, oil, tea, tincture.

Possible Side Effects Can cause photosensitivity in some individuals.

Precautions Parsley should not be ingested in large amounts or used externally during pregnancy; it contains compounds that may stimulate uterine muscles and possibly cause miscarriage.

PIPER METHYSTICUM
Kava

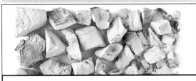

Properties Antidepressant, antispasmodic, aphrodisiac, diuretic, muscle relaxant, sedative.

Target Ailments Anxiety, colds, depression, menstrual conditions, muscle cramps, respiratory tract conditions, stress.

Available Forms Capsule, dried herb, liquid extract, tea, tincture.

Possible Side Effects Allergic skin reactions, muscle weakness, red eyes, sleepiness.

Precautions In high doses, kava can impair motor reflexes and cause breathing problems.

ROSMARINUS OFFICINALI
Rosemary

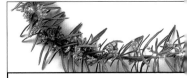

Properties Antibacterial, antidepressant, anti-inflammatory, antiseptic, carminative, circulatory stimulant.

Target Ailments Bad breath, dandruff, depression, eczema, headaches, indigestion, joint inflammation, mouth and throat infection muscle pain, psoriasis, rheumatoid arthritis.

Available Forms Dried herb, fresh herb, ingestible rosemary-flavoured oil, oil, ointment, tea, tincture.

Possible Side Effects Rosemary oil can caus skin inflammation and/or dermatitis.

Precautions Do not mistake regular rosemar oil for ingestible rosemary-flavoured oil.

SILYBUM
Milk Thistle

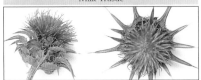

Properties Anti-inflammatory, antioxidant, digestive aid, immune-system stimulant.

Target Ailments Inflammation of the gall-bladder duct, hepatitis, liver conditions, poisoning from ingestion of the death cup mushroom, psoriasis.

Available Forms Capsule, dried herb, fresh herb, powder, tea, tincture.

Possible Side Effects Milk thistle can cause mild diarrhoea when taken in large doses.

Precautions If you think you have a liver disorder, seek medical advice before taking this herb.

TANACETUM PARTHENIUM
Feverfew

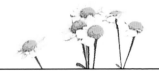

Properties Anti-inflammatory, fever reducer.

Target Ailments Arthritis, asthma, dermatitis menstrual pain, migraines.

Available Forms Capsule, dried herb, fresh herb, liquid extract, tincture.

Possible Side Effects Some individuals experience "withdrawal" symptoms after taking feverfew, including fatigue and nervousness.

Precautions Because it is related to ragweed, individuals with ragweed allergies should consult a doctor before using feverfew.

SALVIA SPP
Sage

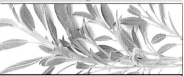

Properties Antiseptic, anti-inflammatory, antioxidant, antispasmodic, astringent, bile stimulant, carminative, reduces perspiration.

Target Ailments Excess intestinal gas, insect bites, menopausal night sweats, poor circulation, reduces milk flow at weaning, sore throat, stomachaches, mouth ulcers.

Available Forms Capsule, dried herb, fresh herb, liquid extract, oil, tincture.

Possible Side Effects Sage tea may cause inflammation of the lips and/or tongue in some individuals.

Precautions Do not ingest pure sage oil; it is toxic when taken internally.

SERENOA REPENS
Saw Palmetto

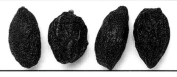

Properties Antiallergenic, anti-inflammatory, diuretic, immune-boosting.

Target Ailments Asthma, benign prostatic hyperplasia, bronchitis, colds, cystitis, impotence, male infertility, nasal congestion, sinus conditions, sore throats.

Available Forms Capsule, dried herb, fresh herb, liquid extract, oil, tea, tincture.

Possible Side Effects Can cause diarrhoea if taken in large doses.

Precautions Due to its hormonal actions, saw palmetto may interact negatively with prostate medicines or hormonal treatments such as oestrogen replacement therapy, possibly cancelling out their effectiveness.

VALERIANA OFFICINALIS
Valerian

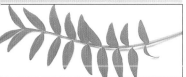

Properties Analgesic, antibacterial, antispasmodic, carminative, reduces blood pressure, sedative, tranquilizer.

Target Ailments Brachial spasm, high blood pressure, insomnia, palpitations, menstrual pain, migraines, muscle cramps, nervousness, tension headaches, wounds.

Available Forms Capsules, dried herb, liquid extract, oil, teas, tincture.

Possible Side Effects Headaches with prolonged use.

Precautions Do not take with other sedatives, including alcohol. Do not drive or operate machinery after taking valerian.

ZINGIBER OFFICINALE
Ginger

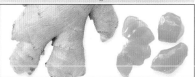

Properties Antibacterial, anticoagulant, antinausea, antispasmodic, antiviral, carminative, digestive aid, expectorant, immune-system stimulant, muscle relaxant.

Target Ailments Burns, colds, flu, high blood pressure, high cholesterol, liver conditions, intestinal gas, menstrual cramps, motion sickness, nausea, stomachaches.

Available Forms Capsule, dried root, tea.

Possible Side Effects Heartburn.

Precautions While ginger is safe in culinary doses, individuals who suffer from a blood-clotting disorder or are on anticoagulant medication should consult a physician before supplementing their diet with the herb.

HERBAL TERMS

ADAPTOGENIC Increases resistance and resilience to stress. Supports adrenal gland functioning.

ALTERATIVE Blood purifier that improves the condition of the blood, improves digestion, and increases the appetite. Used to treat conditions arising from or causing toxicity.

ANALGESIC HERB that relieves pain either by relaxing muscles or reducing pain signals to the brain.

ANTHELMINTIC Destroys or expels intestinal worms.

ANTACID Neutralizes excess stomach and intestinal acids.

ANTIALLERGENIC Inactivates allergenic substances in the body.

ANTIBACTERIAL/ANTIBIOTIC Helps the body fight off harmful bacteria.

ANTIDEPRESSANT Helps maintain emotional stability.

ANTICATARRHAL Eliminates or counteracts the formation of mucus.

ANTICOAGULANT Thins blood and helps prevent blood clots.

ANTIFUNGAL Kills infection-causing fungi.

ANTI-INFLAMMATORY Reduces swelling of the tissues.

ANTI-ITCH Deadens itching sensations.

ANTIMICROBIAL Kills a wide range of harmful bacteria, fungi, and viruses.

ANTIOXIDANT Fights harmful oxidation.

ANTIPYRETIC/FEVER REDUCER Reduces or prevents fever.

ANTISEPTIC External application prevents bacterial growth on skin.

ANTISPASMODIC Prevents or relaxes muscle tension.

ANTIVIRAL Helps the body fight invading viruses.

ASTRINGENT Has a constricting or binding effect. Commonly used to treat haemorrhages, secretions and diarrhoea.

BLOOD COAGULANT Thickens blood and aids in clotting.

CARMINATIVE Relieves gas.

CHOLAGOGUE Encourages the flow of bile into the small intestine.

CIRCULATORY STIMULANT Promotes even and efficient blood circulation.

DEMULCENT Soothing substance, usually mucilage, taken internally to protect injured or inflamed tissues.

DIAPHORETIC Induces sweating.

DIURETIC Increases urine flow.

EMETIC Induces vomiting.

EMMENAGOGUE Promotes menstruation.

EMOLLIE Softens, soothes and protects skin.

EXPECTORANT Assists in expelling mucus from the lungs and throat.

GALACTOGOGUE Increases the secretion of breast milk.

HEMOSTATIC Stops haemorrhaging and encourages blood coagulation.

HEPATIC Tones and strengthens the liver.

HYPOTENSIVE Lowers abnormally elevated blood pressure.

IMMUNE-SYSTEM STIMULANT Strengthens immune system so the body can fight off invading organisms.

LAXATIVE Promotes bowel movements.

LITHOTRIPTIC Helps dissolve urinary and biliary stones.

MUSCLE RELAXANT Loosens tight muscles and reduces muscle cramping.

NERVINE Calms tension.

OXYTOCIC Stimulates uterine contractions.

RUBEFACIENT Increases blood flow at the surface of the skin.

SEDATIVE Quiets the nervous system.

SIALAGOGUE/DIGESTIVE AID Promotes the flow of saliva.

STIMULANT Increases the body's energy.

TONIC Promotes the functions of body systems.

VASOCONSTRICTOR Constricts blood vessels, limiting the amount of blood flowing to a particular area.

VASODILATOR Dilates blood vessels, helping to promote blood flow.

VULNERARY Encourages wound healing by promoting cell growth and repair.

USEFUL ADDRESSES

PROFESSIONAL ASSOCIATIONS

Ayurvedic Living
PO Box 188,
Exeter,
Devon EX4 5AB

British Herbal Medicine Association
Sun House,
Church St,
Stroud GL5 1JL

European Herbal Practitioners Association
Midsummer Cottage,
Nether, Westcote,
Kingham, Oxon OX7 6SD

European Scientific Cooperative for Phytotherapy
Argyll House, Gandy St,
Exeter EX4 3LS

National Institute of Medical Herbalists
56 Longbrook Street,
Exeter EX4 6AH

Register of Chinese Herbal Medicine
PO Box 400
Wembley HA9 9NZ

TRAINING COURSES

Middlesex University
Queensway, Enfield,
Middlesex EN3 4SF

School of Phytotherapy
Bucksteep Manor,
Bodle Street Green,
Nr Hailsham,
East Sussex BN27 4RH

University of Central Lancashire
Preston PR1 2HE

University of Westminster
309 Regent St,
London W1

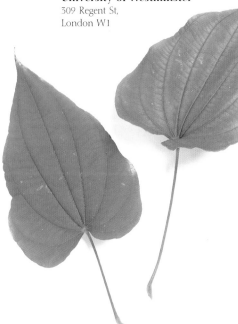